25 RECIPES FOR HAVING A HEALTHY KIDNEY DIET

COPYRIGHT

Table of Contents

INTRODUCTION

If you have renal disease, you can still eat a wide range of tasty and healthful foods. Kidney nutritionists evaluate and approve all of the Kidney Kitchen dishes. Browse our selection of kidney-friendly recipes or use the category filters below.

Components

Any 300g spaghetti shape would do.

400-gram sausages

One chopped leek, one chopped pepper, one chopped tiny courgetti, and one chopped tin (400g) of tomatoes

Crushed garlic clove; 20g grated mozzarella

One teaspoon of dried Italian herb

One teaspoon olive oil

Method

Step 1: Prepare the pasta according to the directions, drain, and set aside. Take your sausages, cut off the skin, and throw them away. Cut each sausage in four, then roll each into a ball.

Step 2: Set oven temperature to 180°C (180°C fan) or gas mark. 4. In a big skillet with heated olive oil, sauté the leeks, pepper, and courgetti for two minutes. After that, add the sausage balls and cook for an additional five minutes.

Step 3: Add the chopped tomatoes from the tin to the pan. Next, pour boiling water into the empty tomato tin, add the garlic, and cook for an additional five minutes.

Step 4: Add the cooked pasta, sausage, and veggies to the pan and stir everything together well.

Step 5: Transfer the mix into an oven-proof dish.

Step 6

Sprinkle with mozzarella and Italian herbs and cook in the oven for 20 minutes. Remove when bubbling and golden and serve into 4 bowls.

The pasta is the main source of carbohydrate in this dish and the value has been provided for those who have been trained in insulin adjustment.

This dish is high in protein and would therefore be suitable for those advised to eat more protein, such as those receiving dialysis. If you have been advised to eat less protein, then you may wish to swap the sausages for a drained 400g tin of lentils.

Use chopped vegetarian sausages (do not create meatballs).

Reduced fat and or reduced salt sausages will make this dish healthier. You may also wish to use whole meal pasta which will increase the fiber content of the dish.

Despite the use of some high potassium ingredients, such as tinned tomatoes, this recipe is low in potassium, when following the quantities in the ingredients, and the serving sizes. Therefore, it is suitable for those advised to lower potassium in their diet.

This recipe is also low in phosphate, however it does contain some phosphate, mainly provided by the sausages; therefore, if you have been prescribed a phosphate binder, you should take as directed.

Use gluten-free sausages and pasta.

Use chopped vegan sausages or a tin of drained lentils and replace the mozzarella with a vegan alternative.

This dish is best eaten fresh.

NaTHaN OUTLaW's FisHGHeTTi

This delicious seafood spaghetti recipe is perfect for weeknights, but great to share with friends at a dinner party too. Using king prawns, scallops and ling or cod, alongside cherry tomatoes and basil. It is every bit a taste of the seaside.

Ingredients

150g king prawns, raw and peeled (approx. 12)

100g scallops (approx. 4)

100g of cod or ling

150ml of tomato juice

200ml fish stock (use low-salt stock if possible)

1 garlic clove

20 cherry tomatoes

350g of spaghetti

75ml of rapeseed oil

10g basil

40g spinach

10g parsley

Black pepper

Method

Step 1: Cut the fish and scallops into pieces of comparable size. It will cook more evenly if you do this. in order for the seafood to cook uniformly, all of its pieces should be of a comparable size. Finely cut the garlic after peeling it, then coarsely chop the parsley and basil.

Step 2: Prepare the fish stock and pour it into a pan with tomato juice. Bring to a simmer over medium heat, and cook for about ten minutes, or until the liquid has reduced by half. Cut the cherry tomatoes in half.

Step Three

While you make the sauce, add the spaghetti to a pan of boiling water and cook according to the package directions. When just cooked, stir occasionally and immediately drain.

Step Four

Add the garlic to a large frying pan with slightly heated oil. Add the fish, prawns, and scallops after the garlic starts to turn color. Fry for 3–4 minutes on low heat.

Step 5: Add the tomato reduction and fish stock to the seafood. Add the spinach, parsley, basil, and cherry tomatoes after that. After two minutes of simmering, turn off the heat.

Step 6: Return the sauce to a low heat when the pasta is done. After adding the spaghetti to the pan and giving it a good stir, season with black pepper. Serve right away.

CARBOHYDRATE

The spaghetti is the main sources of carbohydrate in this recipe and the value has been provided for those who have been trained in insulin adjustment.

PROTEIN

The seafood used in this recipe provides a good source of protein which is great for people receiving dialysis who need to eat more protein. If you have been advised to eat a low protein diet, use a smaller portion of seafood, about third of the recipe portion.

There is no added salt in this recipe, but it is found naturally in the seafood. It is only slightly above the range to be classified a low salt dish. Choose a fish stock cube with the lowest amount of salt.

POTASSIUM PHOSPATE

Although this dish contains some high potassium ingredients, such as tomato juice, cherry tomatoes and spinach, the amounts used are minimal to ensure the entire meal is still low in potassium and can be enjoyed as part of a low potassium diet.

Despite also containing some ingredients high in phosphate, such as prawns and scallops, overall, this dish is low in phosphate and can be enjoyed as part of a low phosphate diet.

This meal still contains some phosphate, so if you have been prescribed a phosphate binder, ensure you take them with this dish.

TUNa PASTA saLaD

This simple tuna pasta salad is delicious and simple to make. Low in potassium, salt and phosphate, it's a good alternative to sandwiches and works well with whole wheat fusilli or penne pasta for added fibre.

A very quick and easy tuna pasta salad that's perfect for lunchboxes and picnics. It can even be prepared the night before!

Ingredients

100g whole wheat pasta, dried

125g broccoli

200g tinned sweetcorn, in water, drained

10 cherry tomatoes (approx.100g)

2 tablespoons mayonnaise

145g tinned tuna, in spring water, drained

Black pepper

1 little gem lettuce

Method

Step 1: Pour half the water into a medium saucepan and heat it up to a boil. Return to the boil after adding the pasta. Simmer, stirring regularly, for 8 minutes, or as directed on the package, or until the food is cooked but still has a slightly hard texture.

Step 2: Prepare the broccoli by chopping it into small pieces. After bringing the pasta and broccoli to a boil, simmer for an additional two minutes.

Step 3

When cooked, pour the pasta and broccoli in to a colander to drain. Then rinse under running water until cool. Drain well and tip into a mixing bowl.

Step 4

Cut the cherry tomatoes in half. Scatter the sweetcorn and tomatoes into the mixing bowl.

Step 5

Using a fork, gently flake the tuna into the salad. Add the mayonnaise, season with black pepper and mix gently until well combined.

Step 6

Serve the pasta salad on a bed of little gem lettuce leaves.

CARBOHYDRATE

The pasta is the main source of carbohydrate in this recipe, and the value has been provided for those who have been trained in insulin adjustment.

PROTEIN

This recipe is high in protein, therefore suitable for those advised to eat more protein, such as those receiving dialysis.

If you have been advised to eat less protein, then you may wish to halve the quantity of tuna. Alternatively, replace the tuna with a small tin of chickpeas (tinned in water and drained). If making this change, the phosphate and potassium would remain low.

WHaT FooDs HeLp KiDNeys RepaiR?

Here are 20 foods that may improve kidney health or prevent it from worsening:

1. Cauliflower

Cauliflower provides many nutrients, including vitamin K, folate, and fiber. It also contains antioxidants and anti-inflammatory compounds.

Try mashed cauliflower in place of potato for a low potassium side dish.

One-half cup or about 62 grams (g) of boiled cauliflower without salt contains:

sodium: 9.3 milligrams (mg)

potassium: 88 mg

phosphorus: 20 mg

protein: 1 g

2. Blueberries

Blueberries are rich in nutrients and antioxidants known as anthocyanins, which may protect against heart disease, diabetes, and other diseases.

They're also low in sodium, phosphorus, and potassium.

One cup (148 g) of fresh blueberries contains:

sodium: 1.5 mg

potassium: 114 mg

phosphorus: 18 mg

protein: 1 g

3. Sea bass

Sea bass is a fish option that provides high quality protein. It also contains healthy fats called omega-3s. Omega-3s may help prevent a range of diseases and boost the health of those living with long-term conditions.

Three ounces (85 g) of cooked sea bass contains:

sodium: 74 mg

potassium: 279 mg

phosphorus: 211 mg

protein: 20 g

However, the National Institute of Diabetes and Digestive and Kidney Diseases (NIDDK)Trusted Source recommends eating small portions of meat or fish, as high protein levels can make the kidneys work harder.

One portion is 2–3 ounces of chicken, fish, or meat, or a piece around the size of a deck of cards.

4. Red grapes

Red grapes are a good source Source of antioxidants called flavonoids, which may help reduce inflammation and protect against heart disease, diabetes, and other health conditions.

One half-cup (75 g) of red grapes contains:

sodium: 1.5 mg

potassium: 144 mg

phosphorus: 15 mg

protein: 0.5 g

5. Egg whites

Egg whites provide a high quality, kidney-friendly source of protein that is low in phosphorus.

Egg whites may be a better choice than whole eggs for people on a renal diet, as egg yolks can be high Source in phosphorus.

Two large, raw egg whites (66 g) contain:

sodium: 110 mg

potassium: 108 mg

phosphorus: 10 mg

protein: 7 g

6. Garlic

Garlic provides a tasty alternative to salt, adding flavor to dishes while also providing nutritional benefits.

It's a good source of manganese and vitamin B6. It also contains sulfur compounds with anti-inflammatory properties.

Three cloves (9 g) of garlic contain:

sodium: 1.5 mg

potassium: 36 mg

phosphorus: 14 mg

protein: 0.5 g

7. Buckwheat

Buckwheat is a whole grain that's low in potassium. It also contains B vitamins, magnesium, iron, and fiber.

It's also gluten-free, making it suitable for people with celiac disease or gluten intolerance.

A half cup (85 g) of buckwheat contains:

sodium: 0.8 mg

potassium: 391 mg

phosphorus: 295 mg

protein: 11 g

8. Olive oil

Olive oil is a healthy source of vitamin E and mostly unsaturated fat. It's also phosphorus-free, making it a suitable option for people with kidney disease.

Most of the fat in olive oil is oleic acid, which has anti-inflammatory properties.

What's more, monounsaturated fats are stable at high temperatures, making olive oil a healthy choice for cooking.

One tablespoon (14 g) of olive oil contains:

sodium: 0.3 mg

potassium: 0.1 mg

phosphorus: 0 mg

protein: 0 g

9. Bulgur

Bulgur is a whole grain wheat product and a kidney-friendly alternative to other whole grains that are higher in potassium and phosphorus.

Bulgur provides B vitamins, magnesium, and iron, as well as plant-based protein and fiber, which is important for digestive health.

A half-cup (70 g) serving of cooked bulgur contains:

sodium: 154 mg

potassium: 48 mg

phosphorus: 28 mg

protein: 2 g

10. Cabbage

Cabbage belongs to the cruciferous vegetable family and provides vitamins, minerals, and antioxidant compounds.

The authors of a 2021 study note that white, green, and red cabbage can help manage blood sugar

reduce the risk of kidney and liver damage

prevent oxidative stress and obesity

A cup (70 g) of shredded savoy cabbage contains:

sodium: 20 mg

potassium: 161 mg

phosphorus: 29 mg

protein: 1.4 g

11. Skinless chicken

Skinless chicken breast has less fat and phosphorus than chicken with the skin on.

One cup (140 g) of cooked, skinless chicken breast contains:

sodium: 104 mg

potassium: 358 mg

phosphorus: 319 mg

protein: 43 g

NIDDK advises people with kidney disease to limit portions of meat and fish to 2–3 ounces, as high protein levels can make your kidneys work harder.

12. Bell peppers

Bell peppers are high in vitamins A and C and other antioxidants but low in potassium.

These nutrients are important for immune function, which is closely linked with kidney disease.

One medium red pepper (100 g) contains:

sodium: less than 2.5 mg

potassium: 213 mg

phosphorus: 27 mg

protein: 1 g

13. Onions

Reducing salt can be challenging, but onions are one way of providing sodium-free flavor to renal diet dishes.

Sautéing onions with garlic, olive oil, and herbs can add flavor to dishes without compromising your kidney health.

Onions provide vitamin C, manganese, and B vitamins, including folate. They also contain prebiotic fibers that help keep your digestive system healthy by feeding beneficial gut bacteria.

One small onion (70 g) contains Source:

sodium: 3 mg

potassium: 102 mg

phosphorus: 20 mg

protein: 0.8 g

14. Arugula

Arugula is a flavorful and nutrient-dense green that is low in potassium, making it a good choice for kidney-friendly salads and side dishes.

Arugula provides vitamin K, manganese, and calcium, all of which are important for bone health.

This nutritious green also contains nitrates, which can lower blood pressure — an important benefit for those with kidney disease.

One cup (20 g) of raw arugula contains:

sodium: 5 mg

potassium: 74 mg

phosphorus: 10 mg

protein: 0.5 g

15. Macadamia nuts

Most nuts are high in phosphorus and are not suitable if you're following a renal diet.

But macadamia nuts are a delicious option for people with kidney problems. They're lower in potassium and phosphorus than peanuts or almonds.

They also provide calcium, healthy fats, folate, magnesium, copper, iron, and manganese.

One ounce (28 g) of macadamia nuts contains:

sodium: 1.4 mg

potassium: 104 mg

phosphorus: 53 mg

protein: 2 g

16. Radish

Radishes are crunchy vegetables that make a nutritious addition to a renal diet. They're very low in potassium and phosphorus but contain other important nutrients, such as folate and vitamin A.

Their peppery taste makes a flavorful addition to low sodium dishes.

A half cup (58 g) of sliced radishes contains:

sodium: 23 mg

potassium: 135 mg

phosphorus: 12 mg

protein: 0.4 g

17. Turnips

Turnips are root vegetables that provide fiber, vitamin C, vitamin B6, and manganese.

They can be roasted or boiled and mashed for a healthy side dish that works well for a renal diet. Alternatively, serve raw, grated turnips with a salad or add them to a winter stew.

A half-cup (80 g) of cooked turnip cubes contains:

sodium: 160 mg

potassium: 159 mg

phosphorus: 22 mg

protein: 1 g

18. Pineapple

Pineapple can make a sweet treat for people with kidney conditions. It's lower in phosphorus, potassium, and sodium than oranges, bananas, or kiwis.

Pineapple is also a good source of fiber and vitamin A, and it contains bromelain, an enzyme that may help reduce inflammation.

One cup (165 g) of pineapple chunks contains:

sodium: 2 mg

potassium: 180 mg

phosphorus: 13 mg

protein: 1 g

How to cut a pineapple

19. Cranberries

Cranberries contain phytonutrients called A-type proanthocyanins. These are antioxidants that may prevent urinary tract and kidney infections by reducing bacteria levels in urine.

Cranberries are also low in potassium, phosphorus, and sodium.

There are close links between urinary tract infections (UTI) and kidney infections, and a UTI can lead to kidney complications.

You can eat cranberries dried, cooked, fresh, or as a juice.

One cup (100 g) of whole, fresh cranberries contains:

sodium: 2 mg

potassium: 80 mg

phosphorus: 11 mg

protein: 0.5 g

20. Shiitake mushrooms

Shiitake mushrooms are a savory ingredient that you can use as a plant-based meat substitute. They're suitable for people with kidney disease who follow a plant-based diet and anyone on a renal diet who needs to limit their protein intake.

They're an excellent source of B vitamins, copper, manganese, and selenium. They also provide a good amount of plant-based protein and dietary fiber.

Shiitake mushrooms are lower in potassium, sodium, and phosphorus than portabella and white button mushrooms, making them a good choice if you're following a renal diet.

One cup (145 g) of cooked shiitake mushroom pieces without added salt contains:

sodium: 6 mg

potassium: 170 mg

phosphorus: 42 mg

protein: 2 g